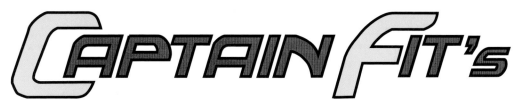

CAPTAIN FIT's
GUIDE TO GOOD HEALTH

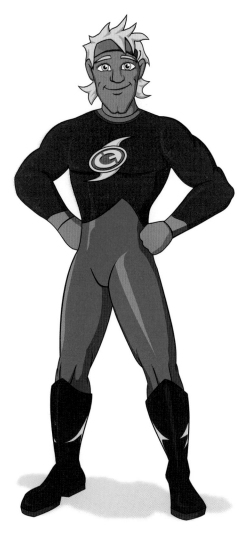

This book is dedicated to all people in need around the world who strive to improve their lives and the lives of their families. Further, this book is dedicated to all those who recognize the value of teaching children good habits for a lifetime of good health. Your children will thank you and Captain Fit™ thanks you. You make our world a better place for all.

About the Author

Matthew E. Alleyne combines his expertise as both a physical trainer and a successful entrepreneur in creating the character of Captain Fit™, and in establishing the Captain Fit Foundation™. His goal is to help children throughout the world improve their physical fitness with a healthy diet, knowledge of personal safety and exercises and other fun activities that can be pursued to develop and maintain physical fitness throughout life. Born in New Zealand, Matthew now lives in Norway with his wife and two young daughters.

Acknowledgements

A very special thank you to my lovely wife, Siw - Helen and daughters, Victoria and Claudia, for their inspiration and invaluable assistance in introducing Captain Fit™ to the world. I would also like to acknowledge the many professionals who helped compile this text and get it ready for your child to read. Finally, I would like to thank the parents and teachers who believe in Captain Fit™ and a healthy lifestyle for children. They make the Captain the valuable resource he is.

Illustrations

The images in this book were created by Sliced Bread Animation, London. To see more, have a peak at www.thebestthingsince.com

ISBN

ISBN-10: 82-997277-2-7
ISBN-13: 978-82-997277-2-3
LCCN: 2005908702

Ordering

To order more copies of this book, and other Captain Fit™ materials, to benefit the Captain Fit Foundation™, please visit us at:

www.CaptainFit.com/store

Your purchase not only helps your children, it also helps children in need all around the globe, and for this, Captain Fit™ thanks you for your generosity and concern for children everywhere. Wholesaler's welcome.

Copyright

Published by Captain Fit AS.
Printed in China.

Meet Captain Fit

Dear Fitness Rangers:

Ever since I was a little captain, I have been on a mission - a mission to make us all healthier and more fit. To this day, I travel around the known universe teaching people, just like you, how to grow strong, how to stay fit and how to make yourself happy by keeping your body healthy.

"My mission is to change the way we eat, and to teach, one and all, the importance of exercise to good health," the Captain said during a recent interview. "Good foods, fun exercise and careful choices - that's what's needed to get fit and stay fit."

The Captain is right. His mission is a noble one. His goal - to help every human being lead a healthier life. Why? "Because a healthy life is a happy life", as the Captain always says. So read on to discover a new world of healthy eating, climbing trees, fun foods, playing sports, lots of easy recipes and tips to keep you safe.

Remember: It's the Captain's mission... but it's YOUR quest!

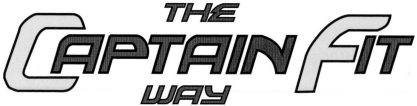

THE CAPTAIN FIT WAY

1. I take charge of my own good health.

2. I eat my vegetables even when I'd rather not.

3. I exercise 20 minutes a day.

4. I only eat junk food on very special occasions.

5. I eat 5 pieces of fruit a day.

6. I eat foods from the four basic food groups daily.

7. I always choose healthy snacks.

8. I never smoke cigarettes.

9. I never use drugs.

10. I never drink alcohol.

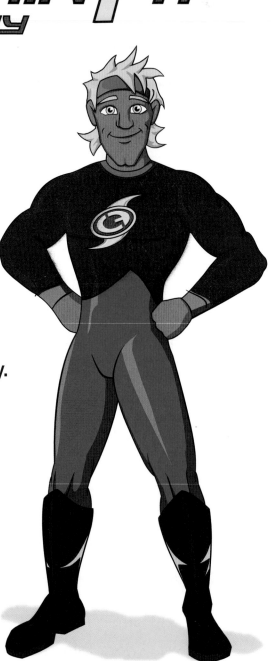

Fun Food Facts, Part 1

1. Did you know that a tomato is actually a fruit and not a vegetable, as most people believe?

2. During your lifetime, you will eat 35 tons of food. Hope you're hungry.

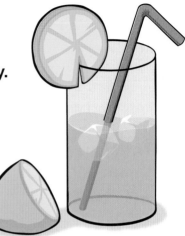

3. Have you ever tasted a fresh lemon? It's so sour it makes your face squoosh up. But how's this for a fun food fact - the sour lemon actually contains more sugar than a sweet, fresh strawberry.

"This lemon contains more sugar than a strawberry"

4. A single, fast-food hamburger can contain more fat than a human should eat over three days.

5. Salt was once so valuable, it was used to pay roman soldiers. In fact, the word salary comes from the ancient roman word for salt.

6. You are much more likely to be hungry on cold, snowy days than on warm, sunny days.

7. Ice cream cones were invented at the St. Louis world's Fair in 1904.

8. Did you know there are over 15,000 varieties of rice?

The Wonders Of The Human Body

The digestive system breaks down the foods you eat so they can be used by your body to maintain good health. Here's how the digestive system works.

1. The first stage of digestion takes place in the mouth. Food is chewed and broken down. Also, special chemicals, called enzymes, start to break down the food before you even swallow.

2. When you do swallow, the food moves down a long, muscular tube called the esophagus. Some people also call this tube the gullet.

3. The esophagus delivers the food to the stomach, where digestion really picks up speed. The stomach churns the food, and strong stomach acids break the food down even further.

"This sandwich goes through a lot of steps before it is digested"

4. Once broken down, the digested food moves on to the small intestine, located just about where the belly button is. In the small intestine, nutrients in the food pass into the blood stream, which carries them to all parts of the body.

5. Food that isn't broken down, or doesn't contain nutrients, passes through the small intestine into the large intestine, sometimes called the colon.

6. This unusable or indigestible food is stored in the colon until it leaves the body through the anus and is flushed down the toilet.

The Digestive System

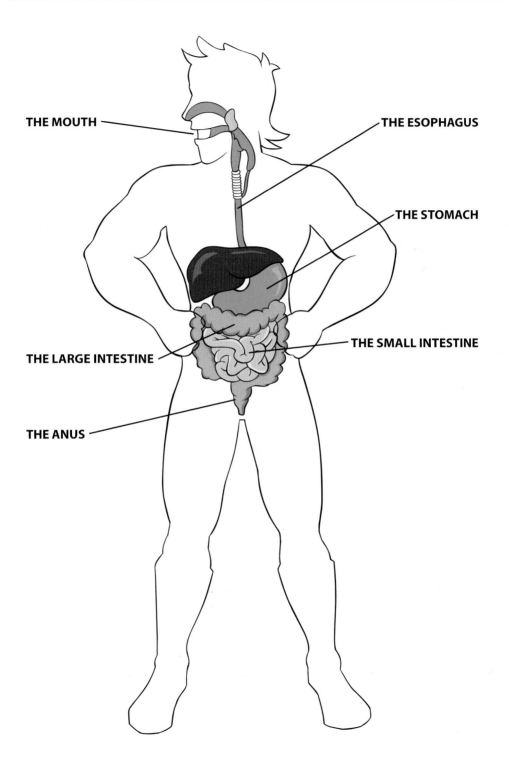

THE MOUTH

THE ESOPHAGUS

THE STOMACH

THE SMALL INTESTINE

THE LARGE INTESTINE

THE ANUS

Tossed Salad, Part 1

Time for a bit of fun with foods, what do you say?

Below are 10 words, but they are all mixed up, just like a nice tossed salad. Can you straighten them out and make words out of these scrambled letters?

Take your time, there's no rush. And, after you have given it your best effort, as you should always do, you can check the answers at the bottom of the page.

So, put your thinking cap on and have some fun with food.

geg ___ ___ ___   epi ___ ___ ___

klim ___ ___ ___ ___   opus ___ ___ ___ ___

febe ___ ___ ___ ___   papel ___ ___ ___ ___ ___

ecka ___ ___ ___ ___   reap ___ ___ ___ ___

west ___ ___ ___ ___   tootap ___ ___ ___ ___ ___ ___

Top Notch Hopscotch

Hopscotch is a fun game, any number can play, you can play almost anywhere and all you need are some stones for markers.

You can make a hopscotch court using chalk on the sidewalk, or make a court in the dust with nothing but your finger.

So, if you've never played, here are the rules to what I call **Top Notch Hopscotch.**

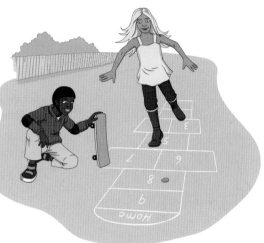

1. The object is to get up and down the hopscotch court, while hopping on one leg.

2. The first player tosses his stone into square number 1. (see above) If the stone slides out of the square, the player misses his turn and the next player throws her stone into square one.

3. Hopping on one leg, she must now jump over square 1 because her stone (marker) is in that box and hop into square 2.

4. In boxes 3 and 4, both feet can come down. Box 5 is a hop, boxes 6 and 7, both feet can come down, boxes 8 and 9 are hops and the half circle is home, where she can land on two feet, turn around and start her way back to box number 2.

5. While standing on one leg, she must pick up her stone marker without falling. She then hops into box 1 and out.

6. You can't step on or touch any lines along the way.

7. If you complete your hopscotch, you then toss your marker into box 2 and repeat, picking up your marker on the way back.

8. You keep going until your stone skips out of a box, you touch the ground with two feet (except where allowed) or you complete all 9 squares.

Facts About Water

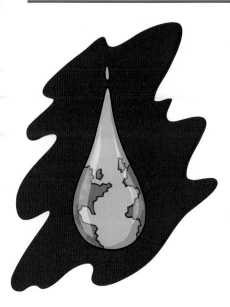

I'm afraid we don't think about water quite enough. Many people don't realize just how important water is. It's an important ingredient in getting fit and staying fit.

I try to drink eight, 8-ounce glasses of fresh drinking water every day. Fitness Rangers should drink between four and six 8-ounce glasses for maximum performance all day through.

Here are some interesting facts about water:

- Three-quarters of the globe is covered with water.

- Only 3% of all water is suitable for drinking.

- The water you drink today has probably been drunk by at least 2 other people some time in the past.

- No 'new' water is made. All that we will ever have is the water that is on the planet now.

- The average person uses more than 80 gallons of water each day.

- Water can be a solid, a liquid or a gas. What is water called when it is a solid? When it is a gas?

- Human beings can live up to a month without food, but not much more than seven days without water. That's how important water is.

- Two-thirds of the human body is made of water. That means, if you weigh 66 pounds, 44 pounds of that is just plain water.

Captain Fit's Tasty Tidbits

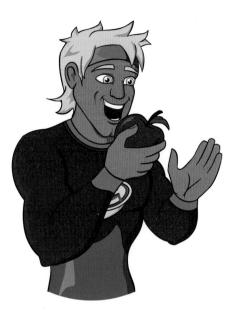

Sure, who doesn't like a nice healthy snack in the afternoon? I know I do. But when I snack, I snack smartly, using the old noodle.

I eat Captain Fit's Tasty Tidbits when I feel a bit rundown. They're snacks that pack a bunch of nutrition and taste good while doing it.

So let me share some of my favorite snack and quick food recipes. They made me the Captain Fit I am today!

Here's a real favorite:

Ants On A Log

One my mom still makes for me, and one you can make all by yourself:

- Wash a fresh piece of celery and dry with a clean towel.

- Stuff the celery with peanut butter, smooth or crunchy.

- Top the peanut butter with raisins. They're the ants on a log.

- Nutritious, delicious and no dirty dishes.

Substitute

Instead of raisins, you can use dried cranberries, fresh applechunks, blueberries or fresh raspberries.

"Use your brain to make your taste buds smile."

Fun With Food, Part 1

Not only are healthy foods fun to eat, they're fun to play with. I'm going to give you three clues, no more, no less. It's your job to guess which food I'm describing. So, let's have some fun with food.

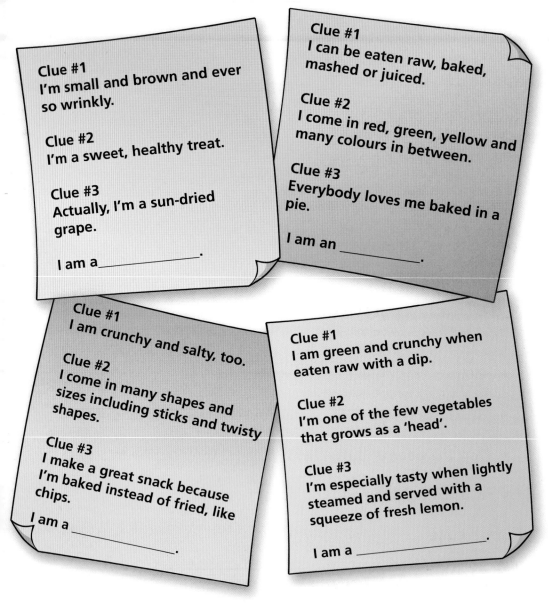

Clue #1
I'm small and brown and ever so wrinkly.

Clue #2
I'm a sweet, healthy treat.

Clue #3
Actually, I'm a sun-dried grape.

I am a _____.

Clue #1
I can be eaten raw, baked, mashed or juiced.

Clue #2
I come in red, green, yellow and many colours in between.

Clue #3
Everybody loves me baked in a pie.

I am an _____.

Clue #1
I am crunchy and salty, too.

Clue #2
I come in many shapes and sizes including sticks and twisty shapes.

Clue #3
I make a great snack because I'm baked instead of fried, like chips.

I am a _____.

Clue #1
I am green and crunchy when eaten raw with a dip.

Clue #2
I'm one of the few vegetables that grows as a 'head'.

Clue #3
I'm especially tasty when lightly steamed and served with a squeeze of fresh lemon.

I am a _____.

Answers: raisin, apple, pretzel, broccoli

Easy Exercises, Part 1

Fitness Rangers, you don't need a special place or time to exercise. You can get a little workout anytime, anywhere.

However, if you haven't been getting much exercise lately, it's very important to start slowly and work your way up.

One of the best exercises you can do when you're just starting out is stretching - stretching out the old muscles.

Here's one stretch that will make you feel good after sitting at your school desk all day, or after a long drive in the car.

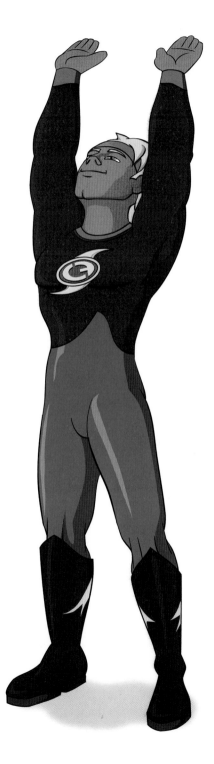

Plant your feet firmly on the ground, toes pointing outward slightly. Then, stand up tall, arms at your side. Slowly raise your arms with the palms of your hands pointing upward. Then, just reach for the sky, slowly stretching the muscles in your legs, back, neck and arms - and that's just about all of them! Try it the next time you're feeling a bit stiff and you'll quickly see how good stretching can be.

Know Your Nutrients

Nutrients are ingredients in food. The human body uses nutrients for many of its activities:

- Healthy body growth

- Daily body repair

- To fight off diseases

- For energy

- Proper running of body systems

Nutrients in foods include:

Protein (PRO-teen)
Used to repair body tissue and to grow muscle

Vitamins (VYT-a-minz)
Used to fight diseases and for the proper running of body systems

Minerals (MIN-ur-awlz)
Used to build bones and the proper running of body systems

Carbohydrates (car-bow-HY-draytes)
Used for energy to stay active and to think clearly

Fats and oils
Used for quick energy

Healthy Habits, Part 1

I always tell Fitness Rangers that good health is not just about what foods you eat, but how you buy those foods, store them, prepare them and save them for leftovers tomorrow. I, and my superhero friends, love leftovers especially leftover soup and stew. They always taste better the next day, don't you think?

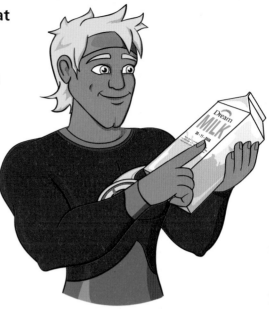

To protect you, your family and friends, here are some important tips on buying safe foods at the grocery store - tips that I follow whenever I go shopping with my mom, Mother Fit.

- Never buy foods that appear to have been opened.

- Never buy foods that look or smell funny or bad.

- When buying fresh fruits and vegetables, make sure they look and feel fresh. Fresh fruits and vegetables should have lots of color and feel firm when given a light squeeze.

- Ask that all sliced meats and cheeses be stored in separate bags.

- Always check the expiration date on items like milk, packaged cheese, yogurt and many other products. Never buy a food that has passed its expiration date.

- When bagging your foods, keep cold and frozen items together to keep them cool until you get home.

- After shopping, don't let foods sit in the car too long. Get them home and into the refrigerator to be safe.

Capture The Flag

Capture the Flag is one of the best games I've ever found. You have to use your brain, your body and teamwork to win this one.

All you need to play is two brightly colored rags. These will be used as the flags of each team. The other thing you need is safe space to play the game.

Here's how.

1. Divide players evenly into two teams.

2. Set the boundaries for game play. ("Over to the big oak and down to the bridge", for example.)

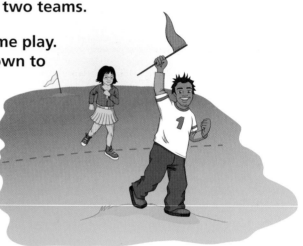

3. Set the dividing line between each team's territory. (The lamp post)

4. Each team then places its flag in plain sight, somewhere in its own territory. You can use team members to guard your team's flag.

5. The object is to capture the other team's flag and return it safely to your territory.

6. If you are in enemy territory, you can be tagged, which means you're caught. You then go to the other team's jail where you have to stay until tagged by a member of your own team. Then, you're back in the game.

7. You can't be caught when you're in your own team's territory.

8. Use scouts to locate the flag, guards to guard the captured members of the other team and the team's fastest runner to make a speedy getaway once you've captured the flag of the other team.

Different Diets

Do you like all of the same foods that your friends like? Probably not. We each like some foods, but not others. Different, healthy people enjoy many different, healthy diets, depending on where they live or what they believe. Here are some of the most interesting diets I've discovered in my travels - all of them will keep you fit as a fiddle.

Vegetarian Diet

Vegetarians don't eat meat or fish. Sometimes, they do this because they don't like the taste of these foods. Other times, people choose to become vegetarians because they don't believe that people should eat other animals.

Since meat and fish provide much of the protein we need to stay healthy and fit, people on a vegetarian diet must find other sources of protein like milk, eggs and cheese.

Vegan Diet

A vegan (VEE-gan) diet has no meat or fish, like a vegetarian diet. In fact, a vegan diet has no animal products at all. No cheese, no milk, no eggs, no yogurt or ice cream.

People who follow a vegan diet believe that we should not use animals as sources of food. Vegans, that's what people on a vegan diet are called, get their protein from soy products, dried peas and beans.

Non-Dairy Diet

Did you know that some people become ill when they drink milk or eat foods made from milk - foods like cheese, yogurt and even ice cream? These people are called lactose (lak-TOES) intolerant. Lactose means milk or from milk.

Since much of the protein in our diets comes from milk and milk products, lactose intolerant people must eat more meat and fish to make up for that lost protein. Many also enjoy 'milk-like' products made from soybeans. These include soy milk, soy ice cream, tofu (TOE-foo) and soy cheese.

The Wonders Of The Human Body

The circulatory system moves blood, bringing oxygen to all parts of the body, while removing waste products produced by the little, tiny cells (SELLZ) that make up everything from skin to hair to lungs and intestines.

1. The heart is the pump that keeps the blood moving. A very, strong muscle, your heart is located in the middle of your chest and a little to the left. If you place your hand there, and stand very still, you can feel your heart beating. It says, 'Lub-glub, lub-glub, lub-glub'.

2. Blood travels through the body in tubes, like water pipes. The largest of these pipes are called aortas (ay-OR-taz), located around the heart. Arteries (AR-tur-eez) are the next largest blood vessels, followed by veins (VAYNZ) and then, the smallest vessels, capillaries (KAP-ih-lair-eez).

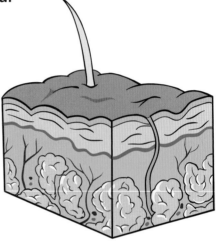

A cross section of human skin seen through a microscope.

3. Blood picks up oxygen from the lungs when you breathe in. The oxygen-filled blood then travels to all parts of the body, delivering the oxygen to body cells.

4. Your heart beats 100,000 times each day. In one year, your heart will beat 36.500.000 times! No wonder a healthy heart is so important to overall good health.

5. Your body contains six quarts of blood (5.6 liters). Each day, the blood in your body travels 12,000 miles (19,000 km) as it moves through the arteries, veins and capillaries.

6. Make a fist. That's about the size of your heart right now. An adult heart is about the size of two human fists.

The Circulatory System

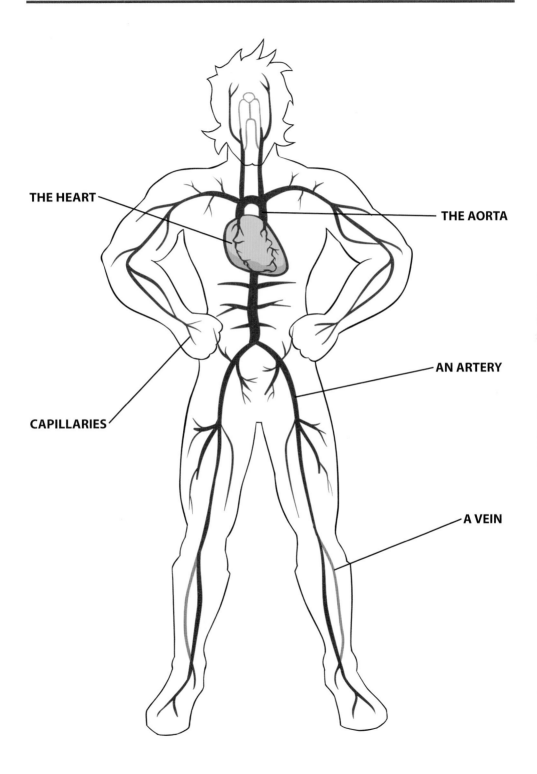

THE HEART

THE AORTA

AN ARTERY

CAPILLARIES

A VEIN

Fun Fitness Facts, Part 1

Being fit is all about eating healthy foods, getting enough exercise and making smart choices about things like smoking, drugs and alcohol. But, being fit is also about fun.

There are lots of stories, myths, legends and other unusual fitness fun from the real world. So take a peek at some of my favorite fitness fun facts to discover just how much fun fitness can be.

Captain Fit

Two Strongmen From Greek Myths:

Hercules (HER- kew-lees) is a hero from Greek mythology. He is remembered for his great strength and bravery. One of the greatest myths is called "The Twelve Labours of Hercules". These labours were great quests and challenges. On one quest, Hercules faced the terrible Hydra, (HIGH-druh) a monster with many heads. Each time Hercules bravely cut off one of the Hydra's heads, two more heads grew in its place. Visit your school or public library to learn more about the amazing adventures of this strong man from long ago times.

Have you ever looked at an atlas? It's a book of maps. The atlas is named after a Greek god named Atlas. **Atlas** was a Titan - a large, strong warrior - who fought against the other Greek gods, called the Olympians, because they lived on Mount Olympus.

The Titans lost the fight against the Olympians, led by Zeus (ZOOSE). As punishment, Atlas was made to keep the earth and the skies apart by carrying a huge pillar to separate the two. In one myth, Hercules takes over for Atlas, but then tricks Atlas into taking up the heavy pillar again.

Easy Exercises, Part 2

You can get a little exercise anytime, anywhere. It doesn't take any extra time and you can do it all on your own. Check out these easy, everyday exercises and put those muscles to good use.

 Don't go looking for the elevator or escalator. Take the stairs whenever you can for a bit of built-in exercise during your day.

 When you do walk up the stairs, take them two at a time. You'll feel your leg muscles grow stronger with every step you climb.

 Walk or ride your bicycle. Don't ask your mom or dad for a ride, ask them for permission! That's right, ask them for permission to walk or ride your bicycle to a friend's house. Not only do you get to visit with your friend, you get a little bonus exercise, to boot.

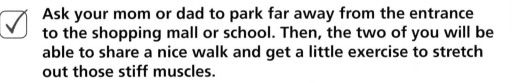 Ask your mom or dad to park far away from the entrance to the shopping mall or school. Then, the two of you will be able to share a nice walk and get a little exercise to stretch out those stiff muscles.

 Don't take a nap, take a hike. If you're feeling a little run down, don't head for the bed, head for the hills instead. A hike through the woods will get your heart beating, your lungs breathing and your spirits soaring - something a nap will never do.

 Do your chores and do them fast. Don't shlump your way through the daily chores. Move your feet, stretch your back, lift your legs and get those chores done faster while getting the exercise you need for good health.

Fun Food Facts, Part 2

1. Did you know that people used to cover a bowl of snow with honey or maple syrup for a wintertime dessert treat?

2. People around the world eat all kinds of foods including snails, rattlesnakes, fried crickets and even chocolate-covered ants. Yummm!

3. Many foods are named after famous people and places.

- The hamburger is named after the city of Hamburg in Germany.

- The sandwich is named after the Earl of Sandwich who enjoyed playing cards so much he didn't want to leave the table. So, he had his servants place meat between bread slices and the sandwich we all love was born.

- Baloney is named after the city of Bologna in Italy.

4. A calorie is a measurement of heat, like a degree on a thermometer.

5. Around the world, hot dogs are called by many different names: frankfurters (after Frankfurt, Germany), franks, hot dogs, dogs, red hots, wieners, weenies, pups and tube steaks.

6. The biggest cookie ever made was a chocolate chip cookie that was 35 feet by 28 feet and seven inches thick. That's the size of a very big room! This titanic taste treat contained more than 3,000,000 chocolate chips.

Captain Fit's Tasty Tidbits

When you're looking for a little snack, do what I do. I stop to think about what I eat, so instead of gobbling down a bag of crisps or a slice of cake, I make good choices for good health.

Here are some of my favorite, quick-time snacks.

Try them, and I'm sure you'll love them as much as I do.

- Spread peanut butter on slices of apple.

- Or, try that apple with a slice of cheese. Delicious and healthy.

- Dip baked pretzels in spicy mustard for a tangy treat.

- Mix granola or cereal into your low-fat yogurt to put a little crunch in your munch.

- Sprinkle raisins or dried cranberries on a green salad, toss with a low fat dressing and enjoy the funtastic flavours of fruits and vegetables together.

- Instead of putting butter on your popcorn, top off this fun time snack with garlic powder, spicy seasoned salt or even a spoonful of brown sugar for your sweet tooth. Mix well, serve and enjoy immediately.

- Freeze fresh grapes for a cool, summertime treat.

Tossed Salad, Part 2

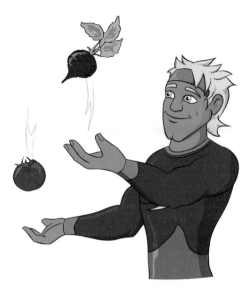

Just in case you forgot how to play Tossed Salad, simply unscramble the mixed up letters that appear below to make some of my all-time favorite foods.

The answers appear at the bottom of the page, but no fair peeking unless you're really stuck.

Now, these might be a little tougher than the first batch, but I think you're up to the job.

So have some fun with food and play a quick game of Tossed Salad.

stota __ __ __ __ __   **grouty** __ __ __ __ __ __

seeche __ __ __ __ __ __   **dalas** __ __ __ __ __

crie __ __ __ __   **cheap** __ __ __ __ __

prage __ __ __ __ __   **shif** __ __ __ __

crator __ __ __ __ __ __   **stapa** __ __ __ __ __

Answers:
toast, yogurt, cheese, salad, rice, peach, grape, fish, carrot, pasta

Funny Food Names

Here's a chance for you to do a little detective work. All of the funny foods listed below are real meals people eat somewhere in the world. Use the encyclopedia, the dictionary or, better yet, your computer to find what these funny foods are all about. Write your descriptions in the spaces provided.

Bubble 'n' Squeak

_____

_____

Toad in the Hole

_____

_____

Shoo-Fly Pie

_____

_____

Bird's Nest Soup

_____

_____

1000-Year-Old Eggs

_____

_____

Hush Puppies

_____

_____

Healthy Habits, Part 2

Time for more healthy habits to keep you growing strong and feeling fit each and every day.

This time, let's talk about how you store foods the safe way - the Captain Fit way.

You might want to mention some of these tips to your mom and dad, especially if they do all of the food wrapping in the house.

The Captain's Food Storage Tips

- Always put cold foods back in the refrigerator after using them.

- Make sure all foods in the refrigerator are stored in air-tight containers, or wrapped well in plastic wrap to keep the freshness in.

- Never thaw frozen foods on the counter. Move them to the refrigerator section the day before you'll need them so they always stay cold.

- Always make sure that beef and chicken are well wrapped and wipe up any meat juices that appear in the refrigerator.

- Store each food item in its own separate container.

- After dinner, don't let those leftovers sit out on the counter. Get them wrapped quickly and back into the fridge so you can enjoy them again tomorrow.

How To Turn Your Backyard Into A Gym

Tag

One player is named 'it'. All players scatter as quickly as they can. The player who is it must then touch (tag) another player who then becomes it. Play this game for 20 minutes a day and you'll be as fit as a fiddle.

Hot Box

You need three players for this game. Two stand on goals set about 20 yards apart. You can use a rock for each goal. The player in the middle must reach one of the goals without being hit by the ball being tossed back and forth by the other two players.

When the middle player is hit, she must stay in the middle. Once she reaches a goal safely, the player guarding that goal takes his place in the middle of the Hot Box.

Jump Rope

You don't need anything but a piece of rope. Couldn't be simpler. You can jump by yourself or with friends if the rope is long enough. The twirlers on the end control the speed of the rope. How fast can you jump?

Soccer Drop

This is an exercise used by soccer players to sharpen their skills. See how many times you can kick a soccer ball into the air without dropping it. It takes a lot of practice, but if you can get up to five kicks, you are excellent. Ten kicks and you're excellent plus.

Hop 'n' Stop

The player who is 'it' turns his back to the other players standing on the start line. He calls out 'Hop, Hop, Hop', changing his rhythm to try to catch players in mid-hop. When caught, they must return to the start line. First player to reach the goal wins.

Fun Fitness Facts, Part 2

Back before television, people used to sit around the campfire and tell tall tales to pass the evening. Each person would make up a story about a character named Paul Bunyan, each more unbelievable than the one told before. Here's a tale tall about ol' Paul's breakfast each morning. Be sure to visit your school or public library to learn more about Paul Bunyan and tall tales. Maybe you can make up your own tall tales. Try it. It's fun!

Paul Bunyan's Breakfast

Paul Bunyan was a mighty man, standing over 20 feet tall before he reached the age of 20. With one swing of his axe, he could fell an acre of forest, and have those trees cleaned of branches before they hit the ground.

Every morning, Paul would eat a hearty breakfast because he knew that breakfast was the most important meal of the day for a lumberjack, particularly one of his impressive size. So the men in Paul's logging camp would get themselves up early to fix Paul Bunyan's breakfast.

A special griddle, the size of a horse corral, was heated. The assistant cook then strapped two sticks of butter onto each foot and skated across the hot griddle until it was as slick as ice.

The flapjack batter for Paul's breakfast was kept in an old water tank, and once the griddle was hot, the cook opened the water tower pipe and out flowed batter as big as swimming pools. Why, it took six men just to flip one of those flapjacks - and ol' Paul could eat a stack of them, you bet.

In one breakfast, that man could eat a dozen flapjacks, 200 fried eggs, 12 loaves of sourdough bread, 18 gallons of cookhouse coffee and top it off with an omelet, if he were so inclined, which he often was.

Only then, would this mountain of a man be ready for a good day's work, and a good day's work is what ol' Paul Bunyan always gave - just like you when you eat a hearty breakfast to start the day.

Captain Fit's Scavenger Hunt

Fitness Rangers, I am sending you on an important mission. This will be a scavenger hunt and you will be the scavengers.

Here are the rules:

1. Each player should have a bag to carry the treasures back home. There are a lot of them.

2. All items must be found within a certain territory. You should not go beyond the boundaries set by your parents.

3. The person who locates all items and returns them to the starting point first is the winner.

4. For larger numbers of players, you can break off into teams of two to get this important task done.

Thank you, one and all, for accepting this important mission.

- Captain Fit

Can You Find These Items Faster Than Your Friends?

- ☑ A book with a red cover
- ☑ Something that belongs to a dog
- ☑ A leaf with notches
- ☑ A leaf without notches
- ☑ Something that begins with the letter M
- ☑ A stone that looks like a face
- ☑ A picture of a flower
- ☑ A real flower
- ☑ Something yellow
- ☑ Something older than you are
- ☑ A piece of fruit
- ☑ Something made of wood

The Wonders Of
The Human Body

When you touch something cold, it feels cold. Touch something hot and - ouch! - it's hot. The human body has five senses: sight, smell, taste, hearing and touch. We can see things, smell what's cooking in the kitchen, taste, hear and touch.

We can do these things thanks to the nervous system of the human body.

The nervous system also moves our muscles when our brains say 'Go' and stops moving those muscles when we say 'Stop'.

That's because the human body is connected by millions of nerves that connect to the brain, which is the centre of the nervous system. The brain receives and sends billions and billions of signals everyday, telling us to do everything from blink to think.

The brain, located inside the head, is connected to bundles of nerve fibers. These bundles run down the spinal cord, located from your neck down through your back.

From the spinal cord, which is a gigantic nerve bundle, smaller nerve fibers spread out from the top of your head to the tip of you toes.

Nerves send pain signals to the brain when you step on a tack. Your brain then sends a signal to your foot to lift up so you don't hurt yourself more. The same with a burn. When you are burned, you feel pain. Instantly, you jerk your hand away from the pain. You don't even have to think about it. It just happens in a wink!

Without a nervous system, we would be cut off from the world.

We would not be able to walk or talk or run in the park. Good nutrition is important to keeping your nervous system working as it should.

The Nervous System

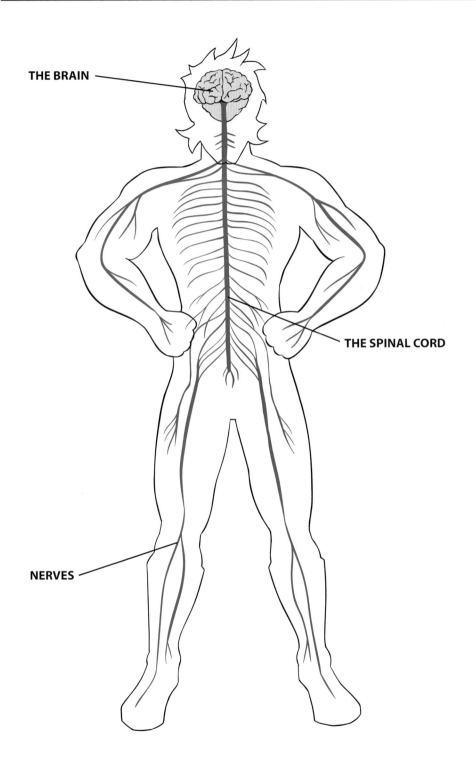

THE BRAIN

THE SPINAL CORD

NERVES

Fun With Food, Part 2

Ready for more Fun With Food. You remember how to play. Just read or listen to the clues to guess what food I'm thinking of. See if you can guess the food after one or two clues to show just how food smart you are. Good luck, Fitness Rangers.

Clue #1
I can be baked, fried, roasted, grilled or microwaved.

Clue #2
I have a brown skin and a white inside.

Clue #3
In some places I'm called a spud.

I am a _____

Clue #1
I am very big and very orange.

Clue #2
I'm best known as a pie filling.

Clue #3
In America, kids paint faces on me.

I am a _____.

Clue #1
I am long and thin and round.

Clue #2
I am boiled when I'm cooked.

Clue #3
I'm often served with tomato sauce and grated cheese.

I am _____.

Clue #1
I am a yellow fruit.

Clue #2
I must be peeled to be eaten.

Clue #3
Many people like me sliced on their breakfast cereal.

I am a _____.

Answers: potato, pumpkin, spaghetti, banana

From The Desk Of Captain Fit

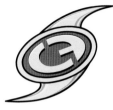

Dear Fitness Rangers

I have received many letters and e-mails from friends just like you. These friends tell me just how hard it is to stay away from those sugary, high-fat snacks.

I, Captain Fit, must admit that I enjoy these foods once in a while. They do taste good. However, they aren't good for your good health.

Below are some of the foods I substitute when I get hungry for an unhealthy snack.

I want all of you Fitness Rangers to start thinking about the foods you substitute healthier choices for your favorite fatty, sugary snacks.

Your friend and fitness leader,

Captain Fit

Captain Fit's Substitute List

Unhealthy Snacks	Healthier Substitutes
Ice cream	Ice milk, juice pops, frozen grapes
Fried crisps and chips	Pretzels, baked taco chips, whole grain crackers, popcorn
Candy	Raisins and other dried fruits
Soda	Fruit juice mixed with seltzer
Hamburger	Fresh tomato sandwich

Captain Fit's Tasty Tidbits

Do you like pizza? I sure do. Too bad it's so fattening. That's why I invented Captain Fit's Pizza With Pizzazz.

Captain Fit's Pizza With Pizzazz

1 tortilla
1/8 cup of crushed tomatoes
1/8 cup of shredded cheese
(the fresh kind)
Sliced tomatoes
Sliced peppers (optional)
Sliced onions (optional)
A teaspoon of olive oil

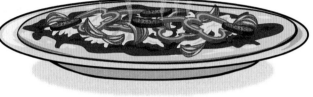

1. Place the tortilla on a baking sheet. Place one teaspoon of olive oil on the tortilla and spread it to the edges until the tortilla is coated with a thin layer.

2. Place the crushed tomatoes on top of the olive oil and spread evenly.

3. Evenly place the shredded cheese on top of the crushed tomatoes.

4. Top with slices of fresh tomato.

5. Add other toppings like sliced green peppers, onions, mushrooms, even chopped up broccoli or spinach.

6. Bake at 350° (F) until the cheese is melted and browned.

Captain Fit's Safety Kit

Fitness Rangers:

From scrapes and scratches to cuts and burns, there are dangers all around the house. It's just wise to be ready for any injury, no matter how small. After all, it's tough to be fit if you're hurting a bit.

That's why I want you to check your first aid kit at home. Make sure you have everything you're going to need in case of an emergency.

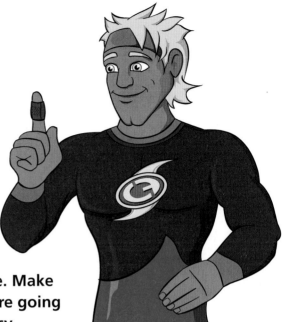

Talk to your mom and dad about first aid and home safety. Playing it safe is the Captain Fit way.

✚ Do you have in your home: | CHKD ✓

An assortment of band-aids	Anti-bacterial ointment
Gauze bandages	Medical tape
A thermometer	Disposable ice packs
Ibuprophen for children	A heating pad (for strains)
Calamine lotion (for itches)	Rubbing alcohol

Dodgeball - Captain Fit Style

This is still my favorite game, Fitness Rangers, and you can play it just about anywhere.

Dodgeball for Two

All you need is a long wall, like the side of a house, and a large rubber ball. One player, called 'the thrower', steps off 10 paces (20 feet) and draws a line in the sand, or uses something to mark the 'throwing' line. The thrower can not cross that line when making a toss.

Player number two stands in front of the wall. The thrower tries to toss the ball to hit any part of the other player's body. If the other player is hit, she becomes the thrower.

Another way we play this game goes like this. Each player gets 10 tosses. The player who hits the other player the most out of 10 wins.

Dodgeball for Twenty

Great for birthday parties, or anytime you've got a group of friends around.

Divide all players evenly into two lines about 20 feet apart. One person is selected to be 'it'. That player stands between the two lines of throwers, trying to get out of the way of the ball being tossed between lines.

When the player is hit, he takes the place of the thrower and the thrower takes his place between lines. Whoever stays in the middle the longest without being hit wins.

Captain Fit's Dodgeball Tip

Most young dodgeball players think that throwing hard is how to win, but I've learned that's not the best way to play the game. Use accuracy, bounce throws and other tricks to fool the player in the middle. If you throw hard, you lose accuracy.

Have A Ball

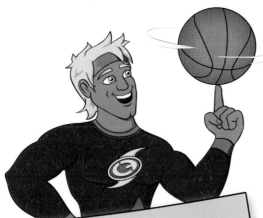

Here's a game that's a real ball - four of them in fact. See how quickly you can guess what kind of sports ball I'm describing from the clues I give!.

Clue #1
I have dimples.

Clue #2
I am small and white.

Clue #3
I am hit by a club off of a tee.

I am _____.

Clue #1
I am fuzzy and come in many bright colours.

Clue #2
I'm hit with a racquet.

Clue #3
Sometimes I get caught in the net.

I am a _____.

Clue #1
I have an orange, knobbly skin.

Clue #2
I am thrown through a hoop.

Clue #3
I must be dribbled.

I am a _____.

Clue #1
I'm a ball that can't be touched with the hands during games.

Clue #2
The object of the game is to kick me into the opponent's goal.

Clue #3
I'm black and white in colour.

I am a _____.

Answers: Golf ball, Tennis ball, Basketball, Soccer ball,

Healthy Habits, Part 3

It's important to prepare foods properly to keep you and your family healthy and fit.

Here are the tips I gave to my own mom about preparing foods safely.

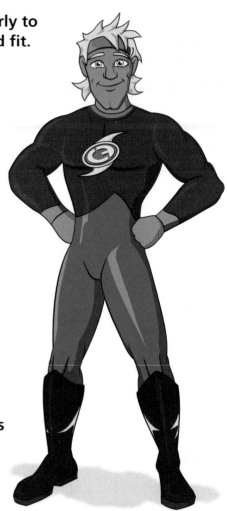

☑ Always wash your hands really well before touching any foods.

☑ Wash all of your fresh fruits and vegetables before snacking.

☑ Use a separate cutting board for vegetables and for meats.

☑ Always wash the cutting knife with soap when working with meats and vegetables.

☑ Be sure to wipe up all meat juices that collect on the cutting board or counter. I recommend using an anti-bacterial soap for this important job.

☑ Carefully follow all cooking directions for the recipe you're using. Never undercook foods like pork or chicken.

☑ Lightly steam fresh vegetables to preserve important vitamins and minerals. Steaming also makes vegetables taste better.

☑ Never use sharp knives, electrical appliances or turn on the stove or oven unless you've received full Ranger training from one of your parents. A well-trained Fitness Ranger is a safe and happy Fitness Ranger.

The Fitness Twist

Here's a mish-mash of words to make you think. Each word is an activity that you can do everyday to build strong bones and muscles. Simply switch the letters around and write your answers in the spaces below. After you've finished this puzzle, choose five of the answers and do each one 10 times before you continue reading.

Get fit, stay fit and have some fun as you do it.

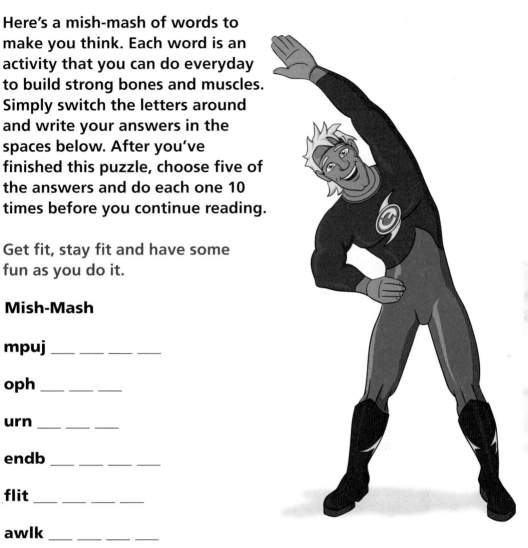

Mish-Mash

mpuj __ __ __ __

oph __ __ __

urn __ __ __

endb __ __ __ __

flit __ __ __ __

awlk __ __ __ __

care __ __ __ __

kips __ __ __ __

pins __ __ __ __

swtit __ __ __ __ __

blmci __ __ __ __ __

caned __ __ __ __ __

worth __ __ __ __ __

chrestt __ __ __ __ __ __ __

The Wonders Of
The Human Body

Your bones are the girders and beams that hold up your body. If we didn't have bones, we'd look like hairy jellyfish. Not very pretty, is it?

Let's bone up on some boney facts, and be sure to take a look at our skinny friend, Mr. Bones Jangles, on the next page to learn the names of just some of the important bones in your body.

- Your muscles hold your bones in place. Muscles also make your bones move when you play or sit or climb a tree.

- The largest bone in your body is called the femur (FEE-mer).

- It connects your knee bone to your hipbone. The smallest bones in your body are inside your ear. They vibrate, making it possible for you to hear.

- Bones connect at joints. Your elbow is a joint where arm bones come together. Your knee is another joint. Can you think of other joints in your body?

- Inside your bones are factories that create red blood cells used to carry oxygen throughout the body.

- When we are born, our bodies have 350 different bones. By the time we're all grown up, the human body has only 206.

- What happened to the rest? They fused with other bones to make one single bone. For example, a baby's skull has many bones, but in time these different bones join together to form a single bone called the cranium (CRAY-nee-um).

The Skeletal System

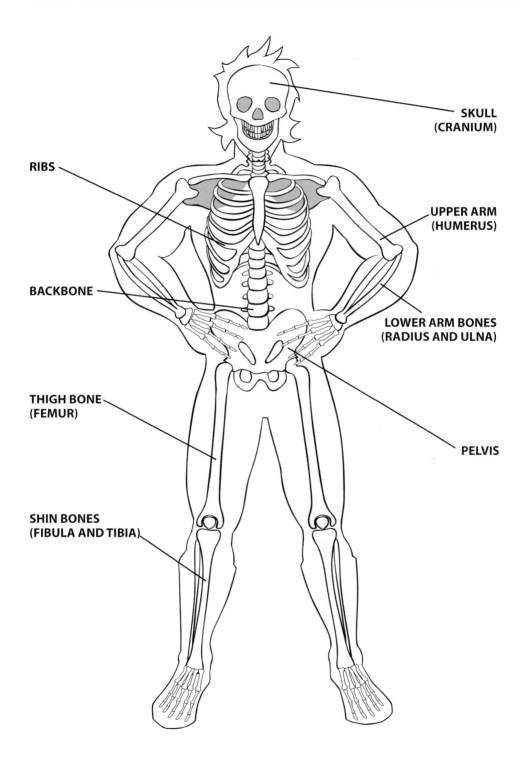

SKULL
(CRANIUM)

RIBS

UPPER ARM
(HUMERUS)

BACKBONE

LOWER ARM BONES
(RADIUS AND ULNA)

THIGH BONE
(FEMUR)

PELVIS

SHIN BONES
(FIBULA AND TIBIA)

The Fitness Rangers' Guide To Fitness

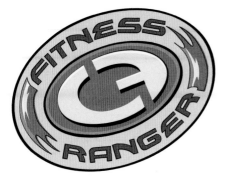

Sure, I know what you're thinking. What's all of this talk about good foods, lots of fresh water and working out, right? Well, we're talking about fitness, Fitness Rangers. Here is how healthy foods and exercise will help you from the top of your head to the tips of your toes.

Fun Exercises Make Your Heart Strong
Your heart is a muscle that pumps blood throughout your body. When you exercise, or just play a game of tag, stop for a moment to feel your heart beating. When your heart beats faster, it beats stronger - and longer.

Good Fitness Will Make You Stronger
When you eat healthy foods that contain a lot of protein, foods like meat, fish and milk, your muscles grow and become stronger. That means that you grow and become stronger.

You'll Be Able To Run, Skip, Hop and Play Longer
Good foods and plenty of exercise build endurance. Endurance is your body's ability to run faster and longer before you run out of energy.

Your Bones Will Grow Stronger
There are big bones and small bones inside the human body. Bones support the muscles and protect your heart and other body organs. To grow strong bones, you need an important mineral called calcium. To get enough calcium each day, drink lots of milk and eat dairy products like yogurt.

Your Body Will Fight Off Colds
Everybody hates colds. You sneeze and wheeze, sniffle and snuffle. When you are fit, and eat plenty of vitamins and minerals, your body can better fight diseases like colds and flu. That means you'll get fewer colds and feel better every day.

Five Fun Activities With Excitement Built Right In

Grab that skateboard
Don't forget your pads and helmet, especially if you're just starting out. Skateboarding is fun, it gets the heart beating and when you catch some air, it's a thrill. I know it is for me!

Skating
It doesn't matter where you skate, or what skates you strap onto your feet. In the winter, enjoy ice skating at the local rink. In the summer, strap on your rollerblades and keep those legs moving.

By the way, try playing hockey on rollerblades. It's fast action and fun to the max. Get some friends together, mark off the goals with some stones, choose up sides and let the games begin.

BMX Racing
Do you think about motocross racing someday when you get a little older? Well, BMX racing is the coolest. You set up your bike, put on the safety gear and wait for the starting whistle. Fast, furious, with just a hint of danger. Just the way I like my sports.

Hiking
I love to hike along the trails, listen to the birds and see the scenery. Look for hiking trails in your area and be sure to take your mom or dad along - or better yet - bring them both. What a great way to spend time with your family.

Snowboarding
Snowboarders are sometimes called shredders, which may tell you something about the way they hit the ski slopes. You can rent a snowboard for the day and even take a lesson. In no time, you'll be shredding up the ski slope yourself - and looking very cool as you do.

Captain Fit's Tasty Tidbits

Like most Fitness Rangers, my favorite part of any meal is dessert. Who doesn't like a nice piece of pie or cake after a good meal? Too bad so many desserts have so many empty calories - calories that don't do your body any good.

Well, dessert time doesn't have to be yuck time. Here are some of my favorite, sweet and tasty dessert treats - treats that provide your body with some nutrients and some fun.

The Captain's Dessert Tortilla

Start with a nice, soft tortilla - the lard free kind. (Lard is a no-no for good fitness.) Drizzle a little honey on the tortilla. Then, sprinkle bits of your favorite fruits - diced apples or peaches or pears, some raisins or other dried fruit. Finally, sprinkle some unsalted, shelled sunflower seeds on top.

Next, carefully roll the tortilla into a tube and place on a microwaveable plate. Zap in the microwave for 1 minute. Carefully remove the plate (watch out, it's hot), wait for your dessert to cool down and enjoy a dessert that's not only good for your taste buds, but good for the rest of you, too.

Mother Fit's Baked Apples

My mom makes these for me, if I ask nicely. Core four baking apples. I like Granny Smiths. Place them in a small baking dish. Pour apple cider over the apples and sprinkle with plenty of cinnamon. Bake for 45 minutes, pouring the juices over the fruit to keep them moist. Let cool. Then serve with a bit of ice cream, or a splash of milk. Good for you and easy to make.

Smoothies

In a blender, mix one small container of yogurt, a sliced banana (or other fruit like blueberries), 1 cup of grape or apple juice, put the top on the blender and blend until smooth and thick. It makes enough for two, so be sure to share.

10 Tips To Save Drips

Fitness Rangers, we all have to do our part to save every drop of water we can. Water is important to good health, but each year we waste billions of gallons of this precious resource. So, here are 10 Captain Fit Tips to save those drips.

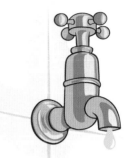

1. When you brush your teeth, don't let the water run. Give your teeth a good brushing morning, noon and night, but turn off the water until you're ready to rinse.

2. Take shorter showers. Get in, get clean, get out.

3. Wash dishes by hand, but don't let the water run as you do. Hand washing uses less water than a dishwasher. Save the dishwasher for really big loads.

4. Never do a half load of laundry. Wait until you have enough for a full load.

5. Place a pitcher of water in the refrigerator. That way, you won't have to run the water to get it cold.

6. Tell mom and dad about dripping faucets. A dripping faucet can waste gallons of water every day.

7. Water the lawn in the early evening to give the grass the most benefit.

8. Help your mom or dad wash the car by hand. It uses less water than the car wash.

9. You can also help mom and dad mulch the gardens. Mulch, like shredded tree bark, helps keep the water from evaporating.

10. Tell your friends. Spread the word about wasting water. Then, they'll tell their friends, and they'll tell their friends, right on down the line.

The Wonders Of The Human Body

We have muscles throughout our bodies. When you wiggle your toes, toe muscles go to work. When you shake your head, muscles in your neck do the work.

Muscles are like rubber bands. They hold in place all of the bones in your body.

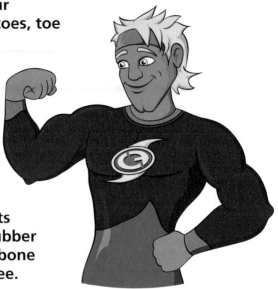

There are different kinds of muscles. Your heart is a special kind of muscle. Ligaments (LIGG-eh-mintz), really strong rubber bands, hold together your shin bone and your thigh bone at your knee.

Muscles stretch and then return to their normal position. When muscles relax they contract (kun-TRAKT). You can tell your muscles what to do just by thinking about it. Go ahead. Wiggle your fingers. See? Your brain told your muscles to wiggle your fingers and they did just that.

Muscles are told what to do when the brain sends a signal through nerves (NURVZ) attached to each muscle, big and small. You think it and your brain and muscles take care of the rest.

Many muscles work without having to think about them. You use muscles to breathe in and out, but you don't have to think about breathing. Little tiny muscles flip your eyelids open and shut when you blink. It's a good thing you don't have to think to blink. You do it 100,000 times each day!

The largest muscle, called the gluteus maximus, runs from your knee to your hip. You use these muscles every time you lift your leg to walk, skip, jump and even hop! The smallest muscles are in your face. These 30 tiny muscles let you smile, frown, laugh, cry and even make funny faces when you want to.

The Muscular System

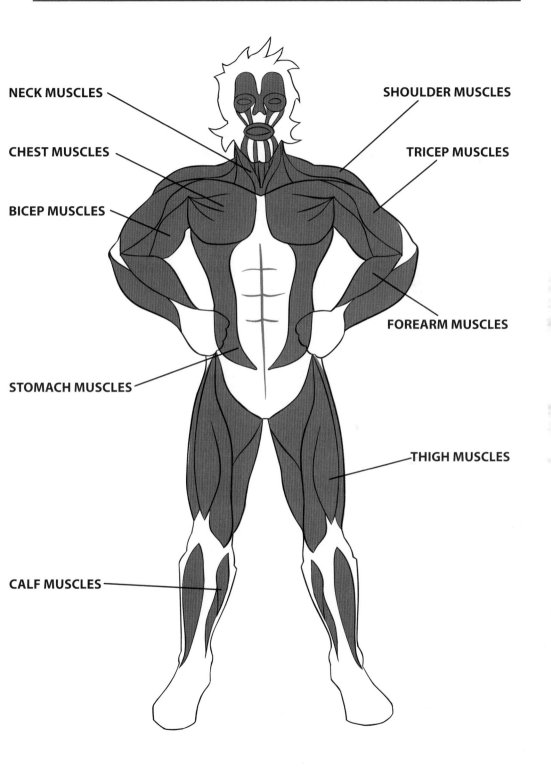

NECK MUSCLES

CHEST MUSCLES

BICEP MUSCLES

STOMACH MUSCLES

CALF MUSCLES

SHOULDER MUSCLES

TRICEP MUSCLES

FOREARM MUSCLES

THIGH MUSCLES

Internet Safety Tips

Your safety is often up to you. Your parents, teachers, neighbours and relatives won't be there all of the time to protect you. So, as a Fitness Ranger, you have to learn to protect yourself.

We all enjoy computer time. We can chat with friends and visit web sites that are full of interesting stuff to see and learn. But computer time can also be dangerous, if you don't take care. So here are some tips to keep you safe when you are surfing the Internet.

1. Never give anyone personal information about you or your family. Never give out your name, address, telephone number, the name of your school or anything thing else. Zip your lip.

2. Never send a picture to someone that you don't know. Never send a picture of yourself or your family, no matter how nice the person might be.

3. Never give out your Internet password to anyone - even to a friend. Your passwords are secret and only you and your parents should know them.

4. Never download anything to your computer without asking permission first. That includes music downloads, too, Fitness Rangers.

5. Tell your parents about any e-mail, instant messages or chat rooms that make you even a little uncomfortable.

6. Always think before you do anything on the Internet. Most people on the Internet are good. Some are not. You can't tell the good guys from the bad guys online, so protect yourself by thinking before you act.

Good Night Sleep Tips

Just the other day, I received an e-mail from a Fitness Ranger asking me how important a good night's sleep is to staying fit. Well, it's mighty important. Many of us just don't get enough sleep at night to keep us going the next day. So, here are some important Captain Fit Good Night Sleep Tips that'll have you rearing to go as soon as the sun comes up.

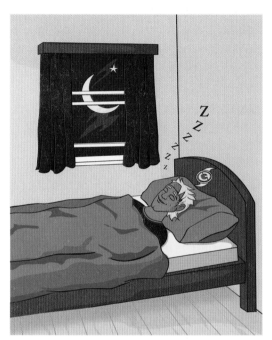

1. Don't eat a lot just before you go to sleep. Eating energizes the body and that's not what you want to do just before bedtime.

2. Don't exercise just before bed. You might think that exercise, or a good game of tag, would make you tired and sleepy. Just the opposite is true. Exercise gives you energy and that makes it hard to fall to sleep.

3. Don't be distracted. Turn off everything in your bedroom. Turn off the TV, the computer, your music and the lights. Good night, Ranger.

4. Go to bed at the same time each night - even on weekends. Your body will fall into a sleep pattern.

5. Open a window just a crack. If your bedroom is stuffy and hot, it's hard to get comfortable for sleep.

6. In bed, lie on your back. Then, starting with your toes, relax your muscles. Relax your ankle muscles then your knees, then your thighs. Relax each part of your body until you reach the top of your head.

Fit Family Vacations

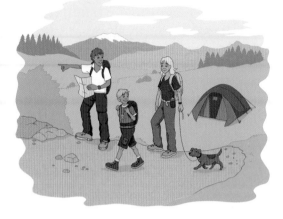

There's nothing better than a fun family vacation, unless it's a fit, fun family vacation.

When I go on vacation, I like to pick places and do things that are not only fun, but keep me in tip-top shape.

So, here are the Captain's Fun Fitness Trip Tips for your next vacation. Drop me a postcard. I'd love to hear from you!

- Ask your mom and dad to pick vacation places where there are lots of different things to do.

- Try a hiking vacation. Each day, you and your family select a different hiking trail to explore. Maybe you can even camp out under the stars.

- Wear the proper clothes. If you're going to spend the day backpacking, make sure to wear your sturdy hiking shoes. Also, pack a sweater or jacket just in case the weather changes.

- Walk. Instead of taking the tour bus, put on some comfortable walking shoes and see the sights on foot.

- Remember your good nutrition habits. When we go on vacation, sometimes we forget about eating the right foods. Remember that good fitness comes from good foods, so eat right to feel right.

- Be careful about the water you drink. Water is different in different places around the world. Before drinking water on vacation, ask for your mom's or dad's permission.

Finding Foods That Fit You

You won't like every food you taste. Maybe you don't like the taste of carrots, or maybe you don't like to eat fish. We all have different 'tastes' when it comes to our foods. The key to keeping fit is to find foods that fit you and your taste buds.

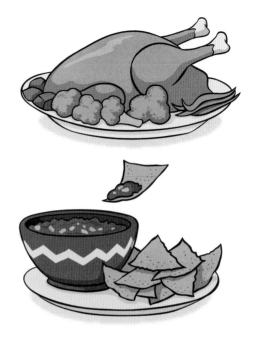

So try a sampling of suggestions from my collection of fit foods that fit you.

1. If you haven't tried it, how do you know whether you like it or not? You can't tell just by looking. Before you say "no" to a new food, give it a taste, a sip or a nibble. You may discover that it's a new food favorite.

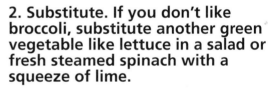

2. Substitute. If you don't like broccoli, substitute another green vegetable like lettuce in a salad or fresh steamed spinach with a squeeze of lime.

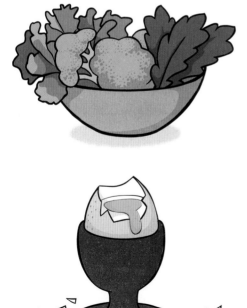

3. Find foods that fit into your life. If you are always on the go, eating a big lunch or dinner may not be the way to go. Instead, have a small lunch and some healthy snacks in the afternoon.

4. Don't eat foods just because your friends do. Maybe your best friend drinks a lot of sugary soda. That doesn't mean you should, or that you have to. Use your common sense and choose for yourself.

5. Finally, keeping fit is something you do every day, not just once in a while. Eat right everyday to find the fit foods that fit you.

Join The Team

There are lots of teams you can join, lots of games you can play. In addition to the good exercise, you'll discover the value of teamwork and you'll make new friends - friends who share the same interests you have.

So take a look at some of the choices you have when it comes to joining the team.

School sports recreational teams

Most schools offer recreational teams for players who want fun more than competition. Here, you'll find fitness, fun and friends all in one place!

Check out the team activities open at your school. You'll find everything from softball to bowling to archery to soccer, without all of the pressure to win, win, win.

Competitive team sports

On the other hand, many people like the pressure to win, win, win. It keeps them going when they get tired or feel down. Most schools offer sports programs in which you play teams from other classes or other schools. It's a lot of fun, but more intense than recreational teams.

Community teams

Ask your mom or dad to check the local newspaper for sports programs in your community. You're likely to find Little League, Youth Hockey, community tennis tournaments and outings to the local community swimming pool. Be sure to bring some friends along to double the fun.

Scouting

Learn to swim, hike through the woods and compete against other scouts. Join a local scout troop, have some fun and get fit while you're at it.

Until We Meet Again

Dear Fitness Rangers

Well, good for you, my friends. You have come a long way in learning about nutrition, exercise and your safety. These are all part of being a Fitness Ranger and you have passed the test by reading this book.

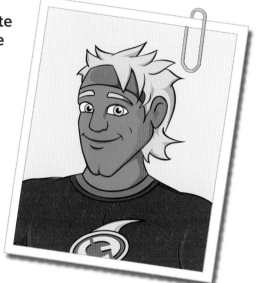

To get you Fitness Ranger Certificate of Excellence, log on to my website and follow the simple directions. That Certificate of Excellence is something you can be proud of. You've earned it because you've learned it.

However, good health doesn't stop here. Now, it's up to you to practice what you have learned. It's up to you to think about the foods you eat and the games you play. Your goal is the same as mine - to spread fitness to every corner of the globe. With your help, we can do it.

Talk to your friends. Instead of staying in to play video games, get out for a game of Capture the Flag. Get all the kids involved. You can do it.

Ask your mom or dad to buy substitute foods for those greasy crisps and chips you enjoy. If you just think about what you eat, you'll automatically eat smarter.

Finally, look for more of my books on how to grow healthy and stay healthy for life. Please visit my web site for the latest news on the latest from the Captain.

Once more, congratulations, Fitness Ranger. Job well done!

Captain Fit

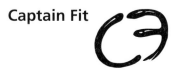

Visit Captain Fit
On The Internet

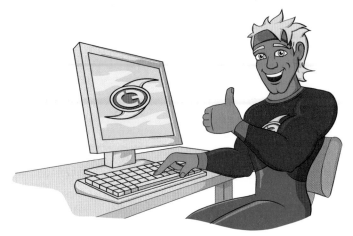

www.CaptainFit.com

There's lots more to discover and lots more to learn about food, fitness and your good health on Captain Fit's web site.

Here you'll find the latest news about all kinds of Captain Fit guides, plenty of tasty, easy-to-make recipes from my own recipe file, games, puzzles and a whole menu of fitness fun.

Become one of Captain Fit's Fitness Rangers to discover even more about growing strong and staying healthy. What does it take to become one of Captain Fit's Fitness Rangers? Well, it's simple. If you want to feel better, look better, think better and be safer, then you're well on your way to becoming a Fitness Ranger.

To receive the Fitness Ranger News and to become a member of the Captain Fit team, ask a parent to signup at the website. Then, just look in your e-mail box once a month for the latest in fitness fun. You'll always discover fitness fun when you visit www.CaptainFit.com.

Hope to see you very soon,

Captain Fit

Captain Fit Foundation

Captain Fit is dedicated to helping people in need all around the world.

The Captain's non-profit organization supports many international charitable groups including: Children International®, Save the Children®, United Nations World Food Program® and the Make-A-Wish Foundation®.

In a recent interview, Captain Fit said, "I help children and parents, not because I have too, but because it's my mission to improve the lives of others, and I want all people to feel the same way."

Your donation to the Captain Fit Foundation™ will make a powerful difference in the lives of others. To lend your support, please purchase our products, or make a monetary contribution directly at www.CaptainFitFoundation.org.

And, from Captain Fit,
a hearty "Thank you, my friends."

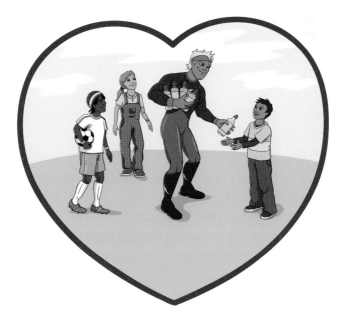

Captain Fit's Recipes

20 great recipes and a meal plan

Just because you need something that's quick and easy for breakfast before school, that doesn't mean breakfast has to be boring. Instead of eating a plain old bowl of cereal, try one of my simple and healthy breakfast recipes. Each one is 100% recommended by Captain Fit.

The Captain's Breakfast Parfait

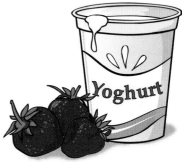

Ingredients:
2 cups non-fat vanilla yogurt
1 cup blueberries
1 cup sliced strawberries
¾ cup Rice Krispies Cereal

Directions:
1) Have an adult slice 1 cup of strawberries before you begin
2) Place 2 tablespoons of yogurt on the bottom of 2 glasses
3) Spread a single layer of strawberries on top of the yogurt
4) Spread a single layer of blueberries over the strawberries
5) Sprinkle 1 ½ tablespoons of cereal over fruit layers
6) Cover with 2 tablespoons of yogurt
7) Repeat steps until glasses are full

Breakfast Banana Split

Ingredients:
1 banana
1 cup yogurt
¼ - ½ cup cereal

Directions:
1) Have an adult help you cut banana lengthwise into 4 pieces
2) Put 4 pieces into a bowl
3) Spoon your favorite flavored yogurt over the banana
4) Top yogurt with you favorite low sugar cereal

FIT TIP: Use cereals that are low in sugar like: corn flakes, wheat flakes or rice puffs.

Captain Fit's Recipes

These two recipes are perfect for those mornings when you're not in a rush. However, for safety sake, always make sure there is an adult around before you start. You may need some help.

Peanut Butter and Jelly Muffins

Ingredients:
3 tablespoons sugar
1 tablespoon baking powder
3/4 cup peanut butter
1 large egg
1 cup low fat or nonfat milk
Your favorite jam or jelly

Directions:
1) Ask an adult for permission to preheat oven to 350° (F)
2) Break the egg into a bowl and use a fork to beat
3) Add peanut butter to the beaten egg and mix with spoon until smooth
4) Add milk to the peanut butter and egg mixture and stir
5) Mix flour, sugar, and baking powder together in a large bowl
6) Pour peanut butter mixture over dry ingredients and mix together
7) Spoon about 2 tablespoons of batter into non-stick muffin tins
8) Top each muffin with 1 teaspoon of jelly or jam
9) Spoon about 2 more tablespoons of batter over jelly
10) Have an adult place muffin tin into the oven and bake for 20 to 25 minutes
11) When the muffins are done ask an adult to remove from oven

Cinnamon and Sugar French Toast

Ingredients:
1 egg
¼ cup low fat or nonfat milk
Dash of vanilla extract
¼ teaspoon cinnamon
¼ teaspoon sugar
2 slices of bread

Directions:
1) Break the egg into medium sized bowl and beat well
2) Add milk, vanilla, cinnamon and sugar to egg and mix well
3) Spray a frying pan or skillet with nonstick cooking spray
4) Have an adult heat the pan on the stove on medium heat
5) Dunk each piece of bread in egg mixture and make sure the bread is totally covered
6) With an adult's help cook the bread in the pan on a low heat until both sides are light brown

Captain Fit's Recipes

Need a way to liven up that boring peanut butter and jelly sandwich? Then try one of these simple recipes that put a twist in one of my old favorites – PB & J.

Waffle Sandwich

Ingredients:
2 frozen waffles
2 tablespoons peanut butter
Your favorite flavor jelly or jam (can substitute with honey)

Directions:
1) Toast waffles until light brown and let them cool for a few minutes
2) Spread peanut butter on one waffle
3) Cover peanut butter with jelly or jam
4) Place second waffle on top of first

FIT TIP: To make this breakfast treat even tastier, choose your favorite flavored waffle. My favorite is blueberry. Just great with peanut butter and Mother Fit's home-made blueberry jam.

Peanut Butter and Banana Burrito

Ingredients:
1 tortilla or sandwich wrap
1 banana
2 teaspoons sunflower seeds
2 tablespoons of peanut butter and honey

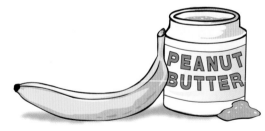

Directions:
1) Spread peanut butter and honey on the tortilla or sandwich wrap
2) Sprinkle the sunflower seeds over peanut butter and honey
3) Have an adult help you cut a banana in half lengthwise
4) Put banana slices on top of seeds
5) Roll up tortilla or sandwich wrap

Captain Fit's Recipes

For those days when I want something a little different for lunch, I make myself either a Southwestern Wrap or a Toasted Tomato and Cheese Sandwich.

Southwestern Wrap

Ingredients:
1 flour tortilla or sandwich wrap
¼ cup low fat cream cheese
¼ cup salsa
2-3 slices of deli turkey or chicken
Lettuce or fresh spinach leaves

Directions:
1) Mix together the cream cheese and salsa until creamy
2) Spread a thin layer of the cream cheese mixture on the tortilla or sandwich wrap
3) Add the slices of deli meat and lettuce or spinach
4) Fold over ends of tortilla or wrap and then roll up

Toasted Tomato and Cheese Sandwich

Ingredients:
2 slices bread or a bagel
3-4 slices of tomato
2 slices low fat cheese
Several spinach leaves (optional)

Directions:
1) Have an adult cut a tomato into 3 or 4 thin slices
2) Place 1 slice of cheese on a slice of bread
3) Cover the cheese with the tomato slices and spinach leaves
4) Place the rest of cheese and the other slice of bread on top of tomato slices
5) Put the sandwich in a toaster oven and set to toast
6) Allow to cook until both sides are brown
7) Ask an adult to remove the sandwich from the toaster oven

FIT TIP: Do you like raw onion slices? Some do and some don't, if you do, add a slice of raw, sweet onion for a lip-smacking treat.

Captain Fit's Recipes

Want to impress your whole family by making lunch or dinner? These two tasty recipes are easy to make and quick. Make sure there is an adult around because you may need a little help.

Tuna Tacos

Ingredients:
1 large can tuna fish in water
2 tablespoons of light mayonnaise
1 package cole slaw mix
Approximately 12 flour tortillas or taco shells
1 or 2 freshly diced tomatoes

Directions:
1) Open and drain tuna fish
2) Mix together tuna, mayonnaise, and cole slaw mix in a large bowl
3) Have an adult dice a tomato
4) Spoon tuna mixture into tortillas and top with tomatoes

Pita Pizza

Ingredients:
Whole-wheat pita breads
Low-fat grated mozzarella cheese
Pizza or tomato sauce
Favorite pizza toppings

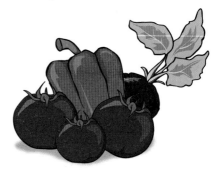

Directions:
1) Ask an adult for permission to preheat the oven to 350° (F)
2) Split the pita bread halfway around the edge
3) Fill each pita with ¼ cup of cheese, 2 tablespoons of sauce and pizza toppings
4) Wrap each pita in aluminum foil
5) Have an adult place the pita pizzas into the oven
6) Bake in oven for 7 to 10 minutes or until cheese melts
7) Have an adult remove the pita pizzas when they are done

FIT TIP: Some of my favorite toppings are mushrooms, green and red peppers, onions, cooked broccoli and cooked spinach.

Captain Fit's Recipes

Spaghetti Pie and Spaghetti Salad are two recipes that my whole family enjoys for dinner. Yours will, too! Check with an adult before you start cooking because you may need some help.

Spaghetti Pie

Ingredients:
6 ounces spaghetti
2 tablespoons butter
2 well beaten eggs
½ cup chopped pepper (optional)

14 ounces pasta sauce
1 cup ricotta cheese
½ cup mozzarella cheese
½ cup grated parmesan cheese

Directions:
1) Ask an adult for permission to preheat oven to 350° (F)
2) Ask an adult to help you cook spaghetti according to directions on box and then drain
3) Have an adult help you chop a pepper
4) Mix together the spaghetti, butter, eggs and parmesan cheese and form into crust in buttered 10 inch pie pan
5) Spread ricotta cheese over spaghetti crust and sprinkle chopped pepper over cheese
6) Pour pasta sauce over pie and have an adult place pie in oven
7) Have an adult remove pie after 20 minutes; sprinkle mozzarella cheese over top and return to oven for another 5 minutes

Spaghetti or Pasta Salad

Ingredients:
1 box spaghetti or your favorite pasta
1 medium sized onion, chopped
½ bottle light Italian dressing
1 medium sized red or green pepper, chopped
1 medium sized chopped tomato
3 or 4 celery stalks, thinly sliced

Directions:
1) Have an adult chop the vegetables
2) Ask an adult to help you cook spaghetti according to directions on box and then drain
3) Pour light Italian dressing over spaghetti and mix in a large bowl
4) Add the vegetables to the spaghetti and mix again
5) Cover the bowl with plastic wrap and place in refrigerator for several hours

Captain Fit's Recipes

An all-time favorite meal around my house is meatloaf. Thanks to my simple recipe, you can make a magnificent meatloaf in just a few minutes.

Captain Fit's Favorite Meatloaf

Ingredients:

1 pound lean ground beef or ground turkey
2/3 cup of low fat or nonfat milk
½ cup bread crumbs

¼ cup ketchup
1 teaspoon salt
1/8 teaspoon black pepper
1 beaten egg

Directions:
1) Ask an adult for permission to preheat oven to 350°(F)
2) Crack egg into a small bowl and beat
3) Place all the ingredients in a large bowl and mix together well
4) Use you hands to form meat into a loaf
5) Place meatloaf in a baking dish or loaf pan
6) Have an adult place pan in oven
7) Cook for about 1 hour and have an adult remove from oven when finished

For a slightly different snack after school or dinner, make yourself a refreshing fruit smoothie. I have one everyday because they taste great and they're great for you.

Banana and Oats Smoothie

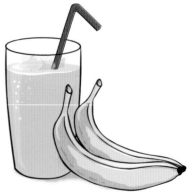

Ingredients:
1 packet regular flavored instant oatmeal
1 cup milk
1 whole banana
1 cup orange juice

Directions:
1) Peel banana and break into chunks
2) Combine all ingredients in a blender
3) Cover and blend on high speed for 1 minute
4) Pour into two 8 ounce glasses

FIT TIP: Out of orange juice? No problem. You can substitute any of your favorite fruit juices. Try apple juice, apple cider or even white grape juice.

Captain Fit's Recipes

Fresh fruit and raw veggies, like carrots and celery, make great snacks. You can make them even better by eating them with one of my easy to make dips.

The Captain's Peanut Butter and Honey Dip

Ingredients:
½ cup smooth or chunk peanut butter
2 tablespoons milk
2 tablespoons honey
1 tablespoon apple juice or water
1/8 teaspoon cinnamon

Directions:
1) Place peanut butter in a small bowl
2) Slowly stir in milk and honey and mix until completely blended
3) Pour in apple juice or water and cinnamon
4) Stir mixture until it is smooth
5) Serve with your favorite fruits, celery, or carrots
6) This recipe makes 4 servings of dip so keep the uneaten portion in refrigerator

Cinnamon Yogurt Dip

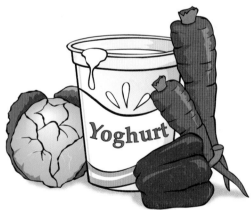

Ingredients:
½ cup plain yogurt
¼ teaspoon cinnamon
¼ teaspoon nutmeg (optional)
¼ teaspoon vanilla extract

Directions:
1) Combine yogurt, cinnamon, nutmeg and vanilla in a small bowl
2) Stir until all the ingredients are blended together
3) Serve with your favorite fruit

Captain Fit's Recipes

Most cakes and pies contain a lot of sugar and other unhealthy things. However, I've invented a couple of treats to satisfy any sweet tooth. And they're good for you, too. My Ice Box Pudding Cake and Mother Fit's Fresh Fruit and Vanilla Pudding Pie are tasty and healthy.

Captain Fit's Ice Box Pudding Cake

Ingredients:
3 ripe bananas
9 or 10 Graham crackers
1 package of instant banana or chocolate pudding

Directions:
1) Prepare instant pudding according to the directions on package
2) Have an adult help you cut the banana into thin slices
3) Line the bottom of a 9 x 9 pan with a layer of Graham crackers
4) Place a layer of the pudding on top of the crackers
5) Add a layer of banana on top of that
6) Continue to layer the three ingredients until pan is full
7) Chill and serve

Mother Fit's Fresh Fruit and Vanilla Pudding Pie

Ingredients:
Fresh blueberries
Fresh sliced strawberries
1 package of instant vanilla pudding
1 ready-made Graham cracker pie shell

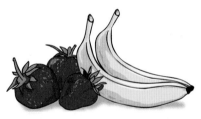

Directions:
1) Prepare instant pudding according to the directions on package
2) Have an adult help you slice several fresh strawberries
3) Place a layer of strawberries and blueberries on the bottom of pie shell
4) Pour pudding into pie shell
5) Cover the top of pudding with layer of strawberries and blueberries
6) Chill and serve

Captain Fit's Recipes

Instead of opening another bag of greasy, unhealthy chips, try making your own using one of my favorite chip recipes. These Pita Chip recipes make a great snack and Mother Fit always serves some with my sandwich.

Cinnamon and Sugar Pita Chips

Ingredients:
2 whole wheat or white pita rounds
Butter flavored cooking spray
1 tablespoon sugar
¼ teaspoon ground cinnamon

Cheese and Garlic Pita Chips

Ingredients:
2 whole wheat or white pita rounds
Olive oil flavored cooking spray
3 tablespoons of grated parmesan cheese
1 teaspoon dried basil leaves
¼ teaspoon garlic powder

Directions for both Pita Chip recipes:
1) Line a baking sheet with foil and get permission to preheat oven to 350° (F)
2) Carefully split each pita bread around the edges so that it forms two pita rounds
3) Ask an adult to help you cut each round into 6 wedges for a total of 24 wedges
4) Place wedges on baking sheet and lightly coat each side with cooking spray
5) Combine sugar and cinnamon together in a small bowl and sprinkle over wedges
6) Have an adult place baking sheet in oven and bake for 12 to 14 minutes
7) Ask an adult to remove baking sheet when wedges are golden brown
8) Let wedges cool completely before eating

FIT TIP: Stay away from fried chips. Go with baked chips and pretzels every time.

	Thursday	Friday	Saturday	Sunday
	1 toasted English muffin w/jam 1 small banana 1 glass fruit juice	1 cup favorite low sugar cereal w/ low fat milk 1 glass fruit juice	Cinnamon and Sugar French Toast 1 glass fruit juice	1 packet instant oatmeal 1 banana 1 glass low fat milk
	Vegetable soup 1 small apple 1 glass water	Waffle Sandwich 1 glass low fat milk	Chicken soup 1 orange 1 glass low fat milk	Ham sandwich 1 glass fruit juice
	Celery or carrot sticks with Peanut Butter and Honey Dip	1 cup low fat fruit yogurt	Graham crackers	1 cup applesauce
	3 to 4 ounce slice meatloaf ¾ cup white rice 1 cup green beans or corn 1 glass water	1 small pork chop 1 cup mixed vegetables 1 small baked potato 1 glass water	3 ounces herb roasted turkey Mashed potatoes Fresh toasted salad w/light salad dressing 1 glass water	Tuna Tacos Fresh tossed salad w/light salad dressing 1 glass water
	3 cups plain popcorn	Any kind of fresh fruit	Small slice of Ice Box Pudding Cake	Fruit with Cinnamon Yogurt Dip

Create your own healthy food plan for a week. Be sure to include three meals each day for seven days, and don't forget those healthy snacks that keep you going morning, noon and night.

Captain Fit's Meal Plan

Planning meals ahead of time is a great way to eat smart and stay healthy. Here's a simple plan I came up with in just a few minutes. Read it over carefully and notice that every meal is a healthy treat.

Meal Plan	Monday	Tuesday	Wednesday
Breakfast	1 packet instant oatmeal Grapes 1 glass low fat milk	1 Breakfast Banana Split ½ glass fruit juice	1 cup favorite low sugar cereal w/ low fat milk Fresh strawberries or blueberries 1 glass fruit juice
Lunch	Peanut Butter and Banana Burrito 1 glass juice	Tuna fish sandwich 1 glass low fat milk	1 Southwestern Wrap 1 glass low fat milk
Afternoon Snack	1 cup low fat fruit yogurt	Banana and Oats Smoothie	Any kind of fresh fruit
Dinner	3 ounces roasted chicken breast 1 baked potato 1 cup cooked carrots 1 glass water	¾ cup of spaghetti w/ ½ cup tomato sauce 1 meatball Fresh tossed salad w/ light salad dressing 1 glass fruit juice or water	3 ounces roast beef Fresh tossed salad w/ light salad dressing 1 small baked sweet potato 1 glass water
Evening snack	3 cups plain popcorn	Sugar free Jell-O	10-12 Cinnamon and Sugar Pita Chips

Spread The Good Word

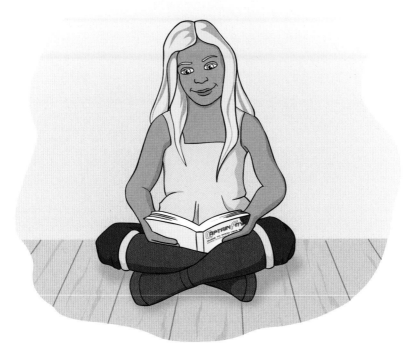

Like you, Fitness Ranger, I'm eager to spread the word about fitness, good foods, exercise and safety. That's why I ask that you share this book with a friend or two to show others that fitness doesn't have to be boring. With Captain Fit, fitness is always fun!

Over and out for now,

Captain Fit